D0254505

HOW TO WEAR

MAKEUP

———

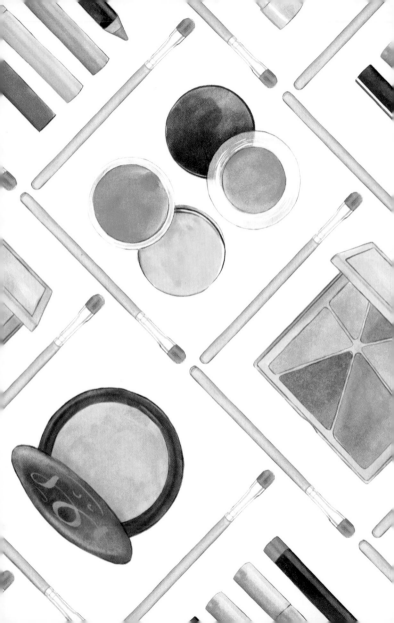

HOW TO WEAR
MAKEUP

———

75 TIPS AND TUTORIALS

Abrams Image
New York

TABLE OF
CONTENTS

INTRODUCTION
6

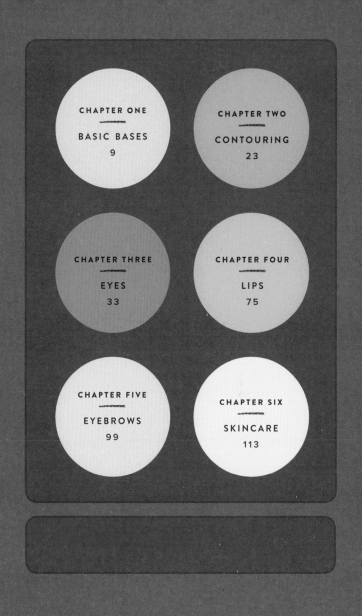

CHAPTER ONE

BASIC BASES
9

CHAPTER TWO

CONTOURING
23

CHAPTER THREE

EYES
33

CHAPTER FOUR

LIPS
75

CHAPTER FIVE

EYEBROWS
99

CHAPTER SIX

SKINCARE
113

INTRODUCTION

A mystery-inducing smudge of smoky eyeliner, an instant-upgrade bolt of crimson lipstick, a cheekbone-sharpening dash of contour powder, a complexion-warming wash of BB cream—the transformative power of makeup has been known to sway mood, seemingly alter bone structure, and make even the most sleep-starved person look well rested.

Makeup's limitless variety of shades, depths, applications, and finishes means that even a single tube of lipstick can be worn in any number of personal permutations. *How to Wear Makeup* is an introduction to exploring the products you already love in new ways and to adding a few future classics to your regimen. In these pages—divided among common colors, exotic executions, and bespoke suggestions—you'll find 75 ways to apply makeup and care for your skin masterfully.

Consider this an invitation to reconsider the contents of your makeup bag and to dip into some more adventurous shades.

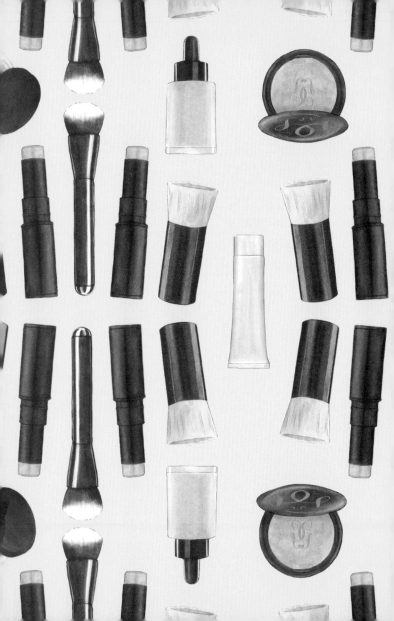

CHAPTER ONE

BASIC BASES

*Complexion perfecting creams
and liquids have the power to take
you from natural to supernatural.
Knowing how to navigate BB
creams, foundations, and beyond
is a lifelong skill, because good skin
never goes out of style.*

CHOOSING A BASE

Whether you're looking for a sheer wash of color or a full complexion overhaul, there's a base for every skin need.

TINTED MOISTURIZER

This straightforward mix of sheer color and moisturizer supplies subtle coverage and hydration to your face. Best for those searching for a discreet pick-me-up for their complexions.

BB CREAM

The BB in BB cream stands for "beauty balm," which marries the benefits of targeted skincare (think: hydration, SPF, and anti-aging properties) with a sheer wash of color. Best for those who want to tint with a focus on prevention and maintenance.

CC CREAM

The CC in CC cream stands for "color correcting," making this product group adept at combating redness or sallowness with, most often, light-diffusing particles and a skin-tone-warming tint. Best for those with uneven complexions looking to conceal existing issues.

FOUNDATION

The most opaque of bases, foundation provides a uniform color to your complexion. Available in sheer, medium, and full-coverage formulas, it's best for those looking to significantly improve their complexions in a pinch, or for anchoring more dramatic makeup looks.

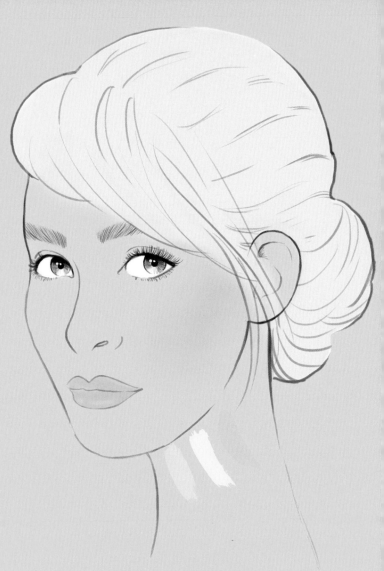

How to
FIND YOUR PERFECT BASE SHADE

A good trick for finding the right shade of base makeup (foundation, tinted moisturizer, etc.) is to match it to the skin tone on your neck. You can also use the back of your hand if you're consistent about wearing sunscreen on your face and are fairer-skinned there than the rest of your body. Leave the product on for a few minutes to see how it adjusts as it is absorbed into your skin. Note that your shades will likely change seasonally with your sun exposure.

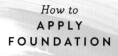

How to
APPLY
FOUNDATION

Using your hands or a large foundation brush, apply a small amount of product to the center of your forehead, cheeks, and chin. Brush the product down to your chin, up to your hairline, and out toward your ears, creating the thinnest layer of coverage at the edges of the face for a seamless transition to your actual skin. If you need more coverage, add slowly. Remember that it's easier to build up coverage than it is to tone it down.

TIP • To blend further, buff over product gently with a kabuki brush or makeup sponge, working in small circles.

TIP • For concentrated coverage under eyes or on blemishes, pat additional product onto problem areas with your fingers.

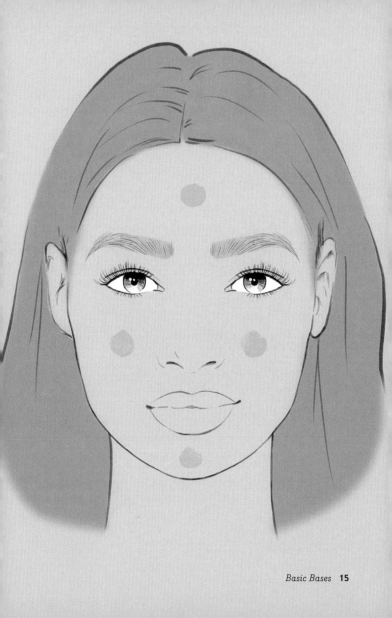

How to
COLOR
CORRECT

Color-correcting makeup camouflages dark circles, sallow complexions, and redness when applied beneath your base or concealer. And they're surprisingly simple to navigate.

PEACH = *Counteract dark circles and dark spots on deep skin tones*

LAVENDER = *Brighten sallow skin*

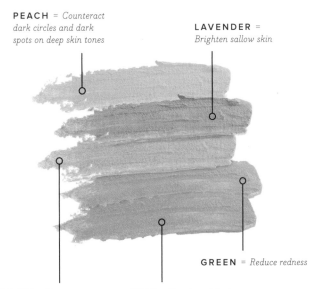

GREEN = *Reduce redness*

YELLOW = *Counteract dark circles and dark spots on medium skin tones, brighten gray complexions*

PINK = *Counteract dark circles and dark spots on fair skin tones*

To cover dark circles, redness, and blemishes, concealer can be applied on clean skin or over foundation.

1

Look straight ahead into the mirror and dab a small amount of product under your eyes, wherever you're dark (this varies from person to person based on the shape of your face and the shape of the space under your eyes). It's better to build up coverage thoughtfully, step back, and add more where you really need it than to put on too much all at once.

> **TIP** • Using a thin concealer under your eyes will help avoid getting pigment stuck in fine lines.

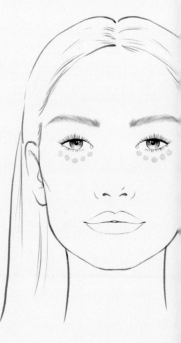

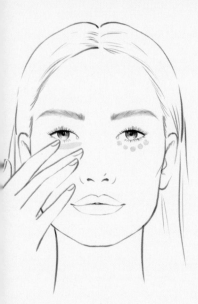

2

Using a small concealer brush or your finger, gently dab and blend the concealer together.

3

Blend the edges into your natural skin tone—be careful to only lighten the dark areas of your face. Adding concealer any lower than your dark areas will cancel out the dark coverage.

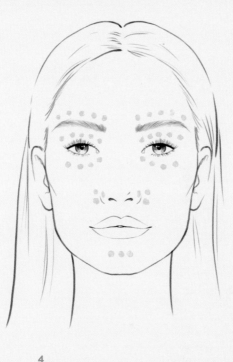

4

Cover areas of hyperpigmentation, red patches around the nose and chin, and blemishes. Be sure to blend edges away seamlessly. Applying concealer just beneath and above the eyebrows will give the appearance of a subtle facelift.

TIP • On the rest of the face, thicker concealers will provide more coverage without the danger of caking up.

How to
USE FACE POWDER

Setting, finishing, and translucent powders are fairly interchangeable products that are designed to mattify areas of excessive shine, blur lines and imperfections, and set makeup for longer-lasting looks.

1

While the product is still closed, turn it over and tap once to release the powder to the surface of the package. Turn the product upright again, and, after opening, swirl a large powder brush to pick up the loose powder.

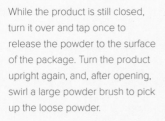

2

Tap the brush to remove any excess product. Then apply the powder in small circular motions onto skin anywhere you want to absorb oil, mainly concentrating on the center of the face (forehead, nose, and chin).

How to
APPLY BRONZER

One of the most misused products in makeup, bronzer is most convincingly employed when limited to the high planes of the face, where the sun naturally hits the skin, rather than applied over the entire face as a universal wash.

Swirl a large bronzer brush into product, tap off excess pigment, and apply the bronzer along the tops of the cheekbones, along the hairline, and down the bridge of the nose. For an extra realistic sun-kissed effect, dab a bit of bronzer onto the chin and along the brow bone.

TIP • The more matte your powder and the cooler the tone (versus a warm tone, which can read as orange on the skin), the more believable it will look.

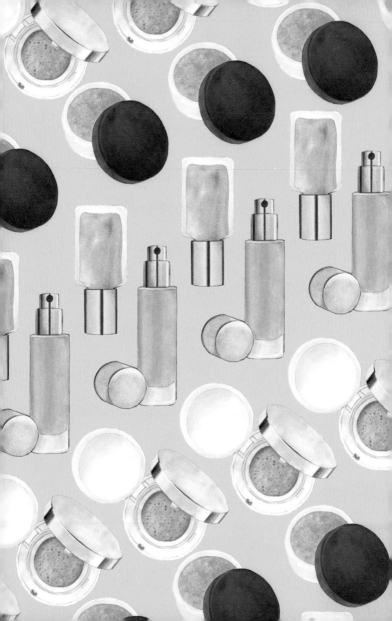

CONTOURING

Enhance your natural bone structure by intensifying the shadows on your face with taupe contouring powders or creams. In other words, create your own lighting.

How to
CONTOUR
YOUR
CHEEKBONES

Razor-sharp cheekbones are no longer reserved for the genetically blessed. A deft application of contouring powder will leave you with lifted, chiseled cheeks.

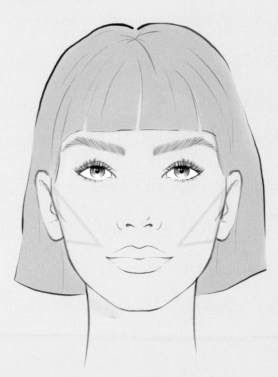

1

Looking in the mirror, gently suck in your cheeks and apply contour product into the hollows with a large contour brush or your fingers—this will typically involve the area on the cheeks just above the mouth and just below the cheekbones. Use a light hand.

2

Blend edges for a seamless finish.

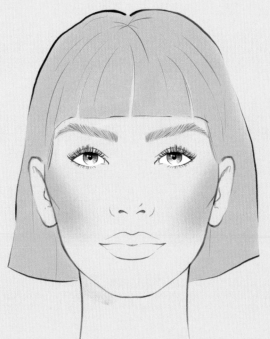

How to
CONTOUR YOUR NOSE

Forgo the nose job; contouring your nose can be used to make it appear slimmer, straighter, and shorter.

1

Starting at the tip of the nose, use a small brush or your finger to draw a highlight along the length of your nose, directly up the center.

2

Starting at the brow bone, use a contour pencil or small contour brush to draw the product down the length of your nose, just to the left and right of the highlight. To visually "shorten" your nose, add a contour just below the tip of the nose.

3

Blend the edges into your natural skin tone.

How to

CONTOUR YOUR FOREHEAD AND CHIN

Contouring the perimeter of your face will help define bone structure.

1

Using a large contour brush or your fingers, apply contour pigment along the hairline, starting at the temples and continuing to the top of the forehead.

2

To define the jawline, start just below the ears and apply pigment along the perimeter of the face and just below the edge of the face, continuing to the center of the chin.

3

Blend the edges of the contour to create a natural shadow.

CHOOSE YOUR PERFECT CONTOUR SHADE

Because contour products are used to create trompe l'oeil shadows on the face, they should be dark and cool in tone, resembling a lack of light.

A good rule of thumb is to choose a cream or powder that is one or two shades darker than your foundation color.

> **TIP** • With a light enough application, even the darkest shades can work on pale skin tones.

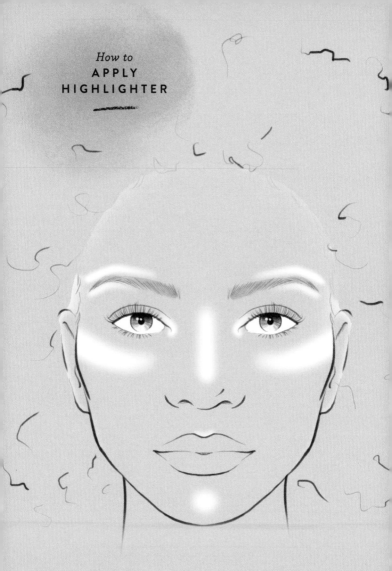

How to
**APPLY
HIGHLIGHTER**

Using highlighter to draw light to the high points of the face is a technique sometimes referred to as "strobing." Like contouring, highlighting helps accentuate your bone structure and can be used in conjunction with contouring or in place of it. Highlighter will also provide a dewy, hydrated finish to your complexion.

TIP • Cool skin tones (including very light and very dark) should reach for icy, white-based highlighters, while warmer skin tones will look more natural with gold-based highlighters.

1

Create a lit-from-within effect by applying highlighter with your fingers to the inner corners of your eyes and to the tops of the cheekbones.

2

Additional highlights can be drawn down the length of the nose, in the Cupid's bow of the lips, and on the center of the chin.

3

Applying highlighter above and below the brow bone will give your face a more lifted look.

How to
WEAR
BLUSH

TIP • When choosing between cream and powder formulas, stick with this golden rule: Powders work best on top of powder bases, creams work best on top of cream or liquid bases.

PALE PEACH BLUSH is wonderful for warming the complexion. When applied between the under-eye circles and the center of the cheekbone, it will draw golden light to your face, and it can also be used as an eye shadow for a bronzer-like effect.

RED BLUSH mimics the effect of blood rushing to your cheeks after coming in from the cold, making you look extra youthful and romantic. For a natural application, concentrate the color on the apples of your cheeks and blend it out toward the hairline and down to about an inch above the jawline.

PLUM BLUSH is especially flattering when applied in a sculpting dash across the cheekbones. Starting at the outer corner of your cheekbone, just higher than the apples of your cheeks, blend the product in toward your nose, extending to the very edge of the hollows of the cheeks.

BRIGHT PINK BLUSH brings life to your face, especially when you're feeling under the weather. Generally speaking, the higher the placement, the more lifted your face will appear. Using the outer corner of the eyebrow as a perimeter marker, apply blush on the tops of the cheeks, below the under-eye circles, and down to the center of the cheeks, directly below the iris. Apply to the sides of your neck for an extra natural finish.

PALE PINK BLUSH is a subtle way to add structure to your face without highlighting. Apply blush between your under-eye circles and the center of your cheekbone, for a natural looking highlight.

> *TIP* • Darker skin tones can layer pale pink blush above bright pink blush for added depth.

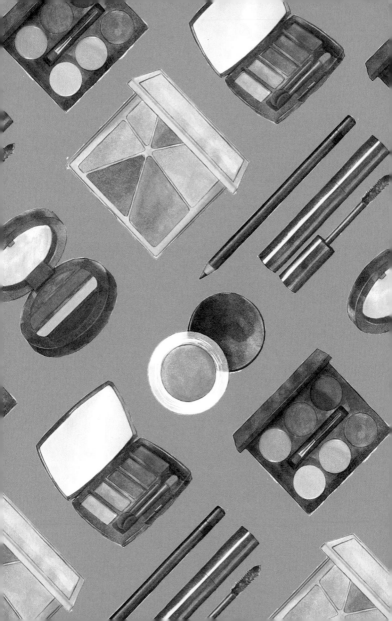

EYES

The windows to the soul, eyes deliver a split-second impression. Liners, shadows, and glosses make it a lasting one.

THE CAT EYE

What do Brigitte Bardot, Sophia Loren, Marilyn Monroe, and Siouxsie Sioux have in common? An angled sweep of eyeliner that has the capability to turn an everywoman into an icon.

1

Starting at the outer corner of your bottom lid, draw an angled line up toward your brow bone at the length of your choosing. This will be the bottom outline of your cat-eye wing.

2

Looking straight ahead, draw a line from the center of your top lash line (just above the iris) up and out to meet the far tip of the first line.

3

Draw a line from the inner corner of the eye to meet the second line just after the iris.

4

Fill in the negative space between the lash line and eyeliner on the inner eyelid.

5

Fill in the negative space between the lash line and eyeliner on the outer part of your eyelid.

6

Curl lashes and apply mascara.

TIP • Felt-tip eyeliners provide the most precision, while liquid liners generally boast lasting power and impact, and kohl liners will provide a smoky, blurred effect.

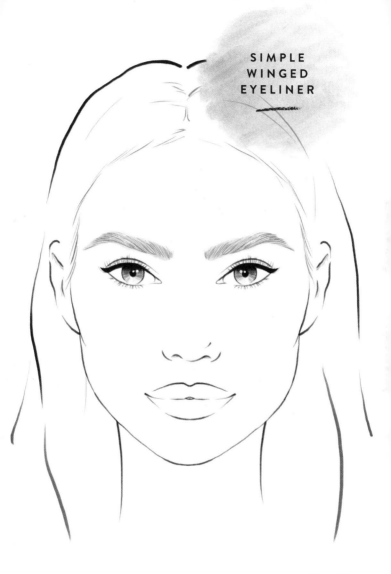

SIMPLE
WINGED
EYELINER

A subtle way to enhance the lash line, a thin swipe of eyeliner will emphasize your natural fringe without the drama of a cat eye.

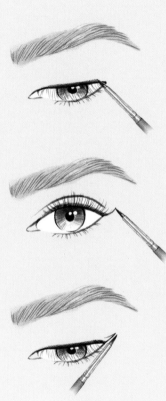

1

Starting at the inner corner your eye, trace the eyeliner as close to your lash line as possible until you reach the outer corner of your eye.

2

Extend the line ever so slightly from the outer corner of your eye.

3

Angle the line up toward your brow bone to the length of your choosing.

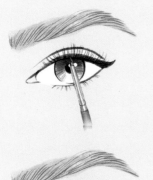

4

Fill in the negative space and any light spaces between your lashes.

5

Curl lashes and apply mascara.

TIGHT LINING

A simple skill for intensifying your eyelashes and eye shape, tight lining can also be used to embolden other makeup looks from a cat eye to a full-blown smoky eye.

1

After washing your hands, gently lift your top lashes upward with your less dominant hand. Draw eyeliner (gel-based pencils work best) along the upper waterline.

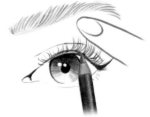

2

Continue the line from the outer corner all the way to the inner corner, filling in between your eyelashes if desired.

3

With your less dominant hand, pull your bottom lashes down and draw eyeliner on the lower waterline from outer corner to inner corner.

TIP • Only tight line the upper lash line for an ultra-subtle no-makeup makeup look.

Beige eyeliner finds its way into makeup bags for its instant ability to fight the effects of fatigue, faking the appearance of a full night's sleep in a single swipe.

BEIGE EYELINER

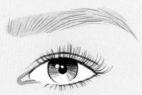

1

Apply beige eyeliner to inner corners of your eye. Blend with fingers if desired.

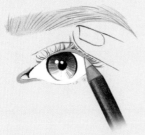

2

OPTIONAL: Tight line the lower lash line with beige eyeliner to make the whites of your eyes look larger.

SLEPT-IN MAKEUP

Since the supermodel era of the nineties, the fashion industry's best faces have sworn that a coat of jet-black mascara and a swipe of kohl look better the next morning. Luckily, you don't have to sleep in your makeup to get a bedroom eye smolder.

1

Using a kohl pencil, draw a solid line from inner corner to outer corner along the top lash line.

2

Stipple dots above the line you've just drawn to create an imperfect, bleeding effect.

3

Using your finger, smudge and blend the line as much as you'd like.

4

Tight line your lower lash waterline with the kohl pencil.

> **TIP** • Concentrate lower lash stippling on the outer corners of the eyes for a wide-eyed look

5

Stipple just below the bottom lashes, creating an imperfect, bleeding effect.

6

Smudge the lower lash eyeliner for a true slept-in look.

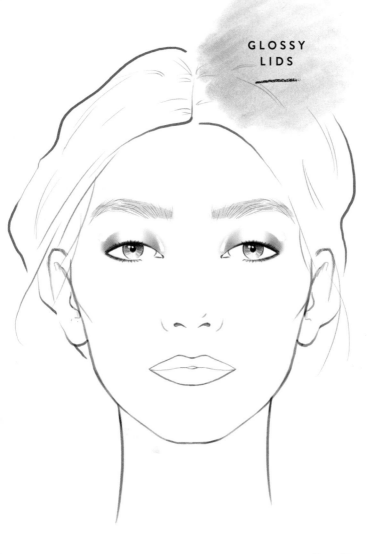

GLOSSY
LIDS

Sexy, dangerous, and fleeting, glossy eyelids are an editorial and runway favorite that seem impossible to execute at home. But only a few products and a laissez-faire attitude about how the look evolves throughout the day are required for real-life wear.

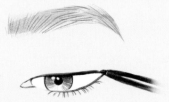

1
——

Start with a thin, lash-defining swipe of black liquid liner from inner corner to the outer corner of your eye.

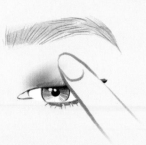

2
——

Stipple a brown kohl pencil along the black line from the center of your eye to the outer corner of your eye, then along the bottom lashes.

3
——

Press a clear, wax-based mixing medium onto the eyelid with your fingers, smudging the brown liner up across the lid and slightly away from the bottom lashes.

4

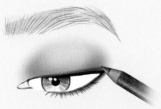

Trace over the brown liner on the top and bottom lash lines with a dark-silver liner or eye shadow, concentrating the pigment on the outer corners of your eyelids.

5

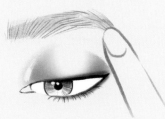

For additional shine, dab a clear gloss on the center of your eyelids if desired.

6

Curl lashes and apply mascara.

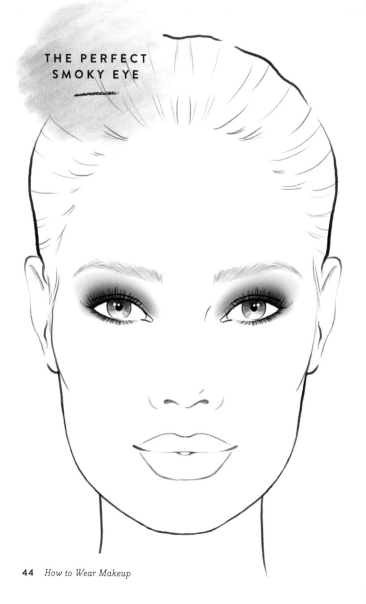

THE PERFECT
SMOKY EYE

The question most often asked to makeup artists, "How do you do a smoky eye?" can be demystified in six straightforward steps.

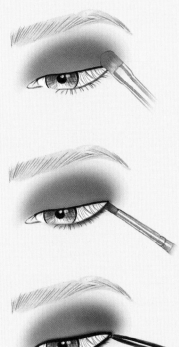

1

Using an eye shadow brush, apply gray eye shadow across the entire eyelid all the way up to the hollow beneath the brow bone and just past the outer corner of the eyelid.

2

Using an eyeliner brush, apply a dark-gray eye shadow along the bottom lash line.

3

Apply black eyeliner to the bottom lash waterline (the strip of skin between your eyelashes and eyes).

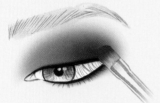

Using an eye shadow brush, concentrate a darker gray shadow on the outer corner of the eye, all the way up to the hollow beneath the brow bone and out to just past the eyelid.

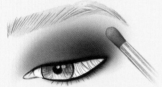

5

Apply black liner to the top lash line, close to the lashes.

6

Curl lashes and apply mascara.

> **TIP** • Try this look in subtle browns for a daytime take on the smoky eye.

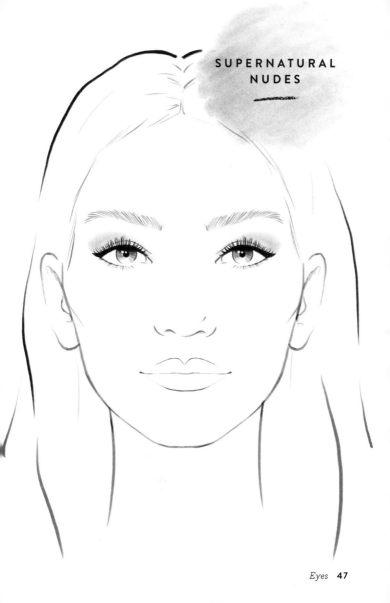

SUPERNATURAL
NUDES

Nude eye shadow gives depth and draws attention to the eyes without showing a trace of makeup.

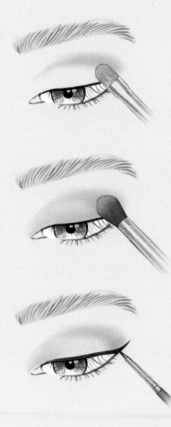

1

Using a shade slightly darker than your own skin tone, apply the nude eye shadow with an eye shadow brush into the banana (crease) of your eyelid.

2

Apply the eye shadow along your top lash line.

3

Blend the color across your lid.

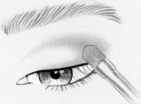

Press highlighter into the inner corners of your eyes and onto the center of your eyelids with your fingers.

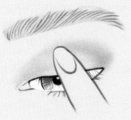

5

To amplify the look, if desired, apply dark brown eyeliner using the simple winged eyeliner technique (see page 35) and tight line (see page 38) the upper lash line.

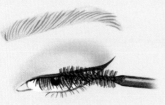

6

Curl eyelashes and apply mascara.

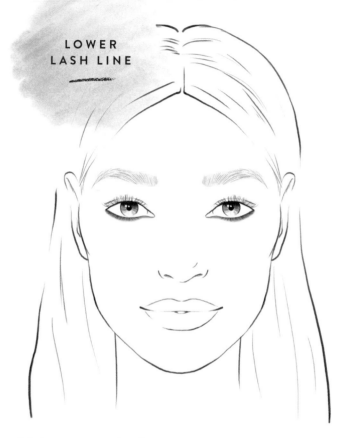

LOWER
LASH LINE

Painting a sooty smudge of pigment along the lower lash line—and nowhere else—makes for a daring, angular, and altogether cool approach to makeup.

Starting at the inner corner, use a kohl pencil or gel eyeliner to draw eyeliner out toward the outer corner of the eye. Smudge with fingers if desired.

THE IMPORTANCE OF AN EYELASH CURLER

With the pinch of a lash curler, your eyes instantly look larger and more awake. No makeup required.

1

Line up the eyelash curler at the base of your lashes, with your lashes between the top and bottom pieces. Clamp down.

2

Gently lift the curler without pulling your lashes for an ultra-curled finish.

MASCARA BASICS

1

To avoid clumps, starting underneath the lashes, place your mascara wand at the root of your lashes and wiggle it side to side.

2

Continue that movement up to the tips of the lashes. Repeat if necessary.

> **TIP** • Make your eyes look wider by concentrating mascara at the outer corners of the eyes. Concentrating the mascara in the center of your lash line will make your eyes look bigger.

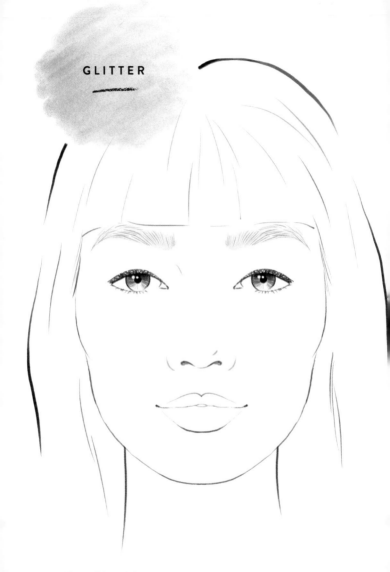

GLITTER

Light-catching glitter is an embellishment that can be taken from the festival to the street—it's only a matter of application.

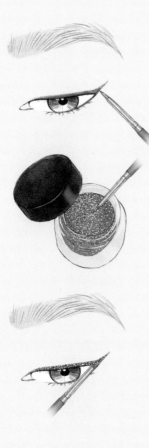

THE MINIMALIST SWOOSH

1

Draw a slim silver cat eye along your top lash line.

2

Dip a thin eyeliner brush in an adhesive (such as a mixing medium or lip gloss) and then dip the brush in loose silver glitter.

3

Paint the glitter across the silver eyeliner on your top eyelid.

4

Add more glitter as desired.

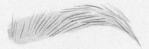

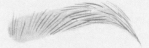

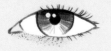

THE LOW-KEY BOTTOM LINER

For subtle embellishment, paint loose glitter along your lower lash line, using a mixing medium as an adhesive.

BORROWED FROM THE BOYS

The most festival-ready glitter application lies in a dusting of the upper cheeks, starting at the eye. It's a look taken from the pages of Shakespearian pixies and glam rock musicians including David Bowie and Marc Bolan.

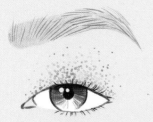 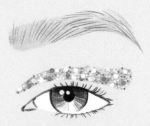

THE BIG SPLASH

Give your makeup a playful disco nod by applying a clear mixing medium or eye gloss to your eyelids, then pressing on as much loose glitter as desired.

THE BOLD STRIPE

Just above the eyelid but just below the brow, a thick strip of chromatic sparkles is at once unexpected and entirely modern.

TIP • The fastest and easiest way to clean up rogue glitter on your face is with masking tape.

BLUE EYE SHADOW 101

Once a vintage remnant of the disco seventies and sock-hop fifties, blue eye shadow is experiencing a modern resurgence by way of bold shades and crisp application.

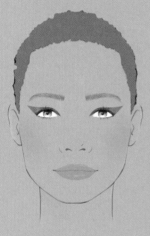

FOREVER IN BLUE COBALT

There's a reason Yves Klein spent a career painting in the purest form of cobalt. Its mesmerizing effects have been proven by ancient Egyptians and modern-day Cleopatras alike.

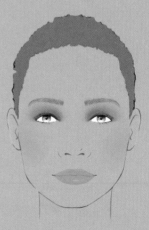

NAVY NIGHTS

The softer side of a smoky eye is no less impactful and universally flattering.

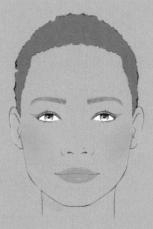

TURQUOISE AMBITION

Intense pigment requires clean shapes for successful execution, no matter your skin tone. An exaggerated cat eye painted opaquely across the entire lid is a surefire knockout.

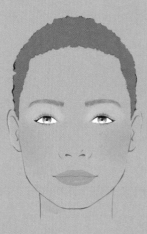

PASTEL DREAMS

A wash of barely-blue matte shadow will bring a charming, powdery pause to dewy complexions.

THE BEST COLORS FOR GREEN EYES

Amplifying the mossy, verdant tones in your iris is as simple as choosing the right eye shadow and liner.

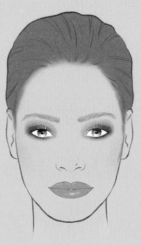

GRAY

The universally flattering tone for the smokiest shadow has an even bigger impact on grassy eyes.

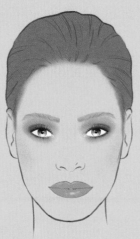

BROWN

As in nature, brown shadow helps green eyes show like leaves against tree bark.

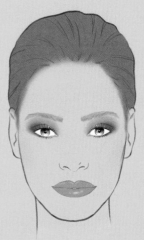

TAUPE

A swirl of earth-tone taupe will draw out the blue tones of your eyes, thus making greens look even greener.

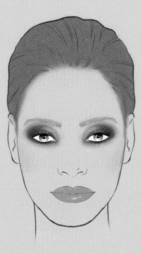

SILVER

Light-catching metallics in cool grays set malachite irises aglow.

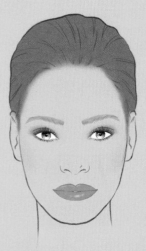

PURPLE

Using the laws of the color wheel, one of green's best complementary colors, purple, will make it pop more than any other shade.

THE BEST COLORS FOR BROWN EYES

The eye color for over half of the world's population can anchor just about any shadow, but certain shades prove ever so slightly more enchanting.

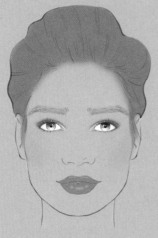

NAVY

The universally flattering shade is especially adept at warming up eye colors from amber to coffee.

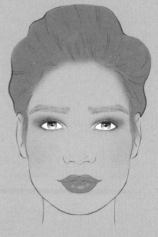

KHAKI

Earthy tones of yellow and green complement their naturally-occurring neighbor, brown, like a slant rhyme.

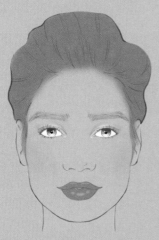

GOLD
One of the most precious naturally occurring metal looks extra bright on dark, deep eyes.

BLUE
Shades of cobalt, sky, and cerulean go together with brown eyes like water and sand.

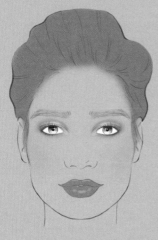

BRONZE
A metallic take on your natural eye color, bronze shadows and liners will cause your irises to shine.

THE BEST COLORS FOR BLUE EYES

From pale and icy to deep indigo, a blue-eyed gaze becomes even more alluring with the help of specialized shades.

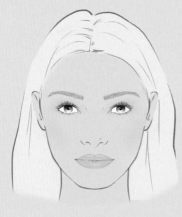

BEIGE
Ecru tones anchor sapphire stares with the slightest definition.

BRONZE
The shimmering sister to orange will draw the most attention to your watery gaze.

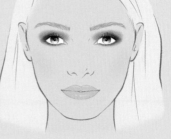

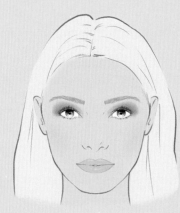

WARM NEUTRALS

Seeing the world through rose-colored eye shadow, blue eyes look especially becoming.

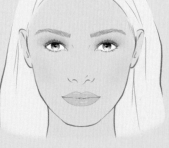

PURPLE

This just-off-blue shade offers a pleasing and subtle color play.

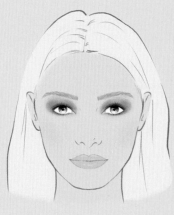

ORANGE

The warmer the shadow, the cooler the iris. Think of a vibrant sun setting on a tranquil, dark ocean.

How to
WEAR
METALLICS

A beguiling way to draw light to the face, go for heavy metals or a barely-there glint.

THE ALL-OVER BRONZE

An eyebrow-to-lower-lash-line rimming of bronze shadow is a graphic and skin tone-warming look ripe for summer nights and winter soirees.

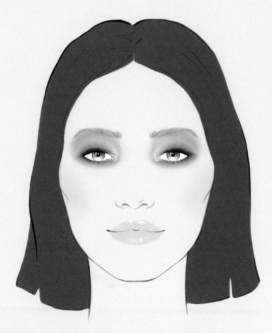

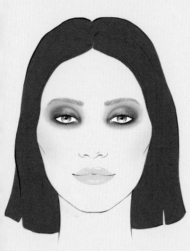

THE METALLIC SMOKY EYE

Using the same principles as a basic smoky eye, painting a bit of copper pigment onto the eyelid and blending out into dark grays and blacks gives a rock 'n' roll appeal to an already glamorous look.

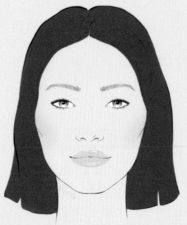

THE NEARLY NUDE

A wash of shimmering peach on darker skin tones and pale gold for lighter shades is a sure and subtle means of brightening your complexion and mood.

THE TWO-TONE LINER

For a mischievous shake-up, try a swipe of silver liner across the top lid and a thin line of gold along the bottom.

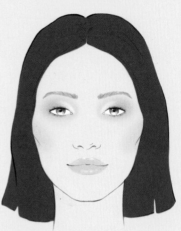

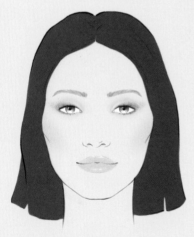

THE GOLDEN EYE

Trade out your black liner in favor of a solid-gold cat eye that will take femme fatale to gleaming new heights.

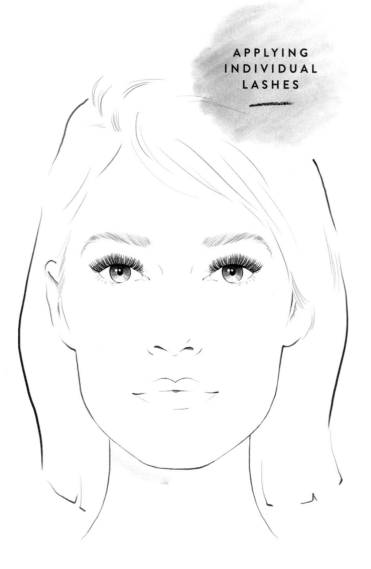

A few doe-like individual lashes will boost the power of your gaze and shave years off your look.

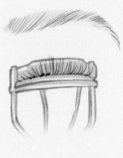

1

Curl your eyelashes.

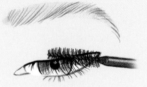

2

Apply mascara.

3

Using tweezers, pick up a single lash from the center of its curve and dip the root into glue.

> **TIP** • Try white eyelash glue that dries clear for easy-to-see application.

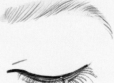
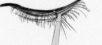

4

Place the fake lash onto your natural lashes, close to the roots, so it is attached to your lashes instead of your skin.

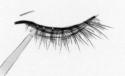

5

Place longer lashes toward the outer corners of the eyes, gradually using shorter lashes as you move toward your nose.

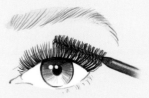
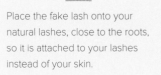

6

Once they are dry, apply mascara for more impact.

> **TIP** • You have around a minute to adjust lashes while they dry.

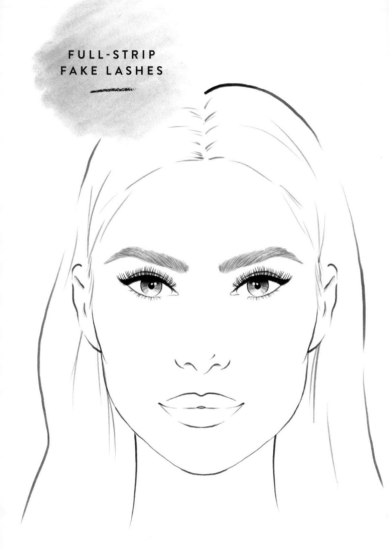

FULL-STRIP
FAKE LASHES

A full strip of lashes can be as subtle or as dramatic as you please, depending on length and material. No matter the impact in mind, a few simple steps will result in a foolproof application.

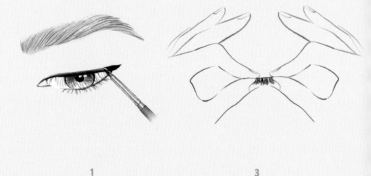

1

Apply a thin line of black eyeliner across the top eyelids, from corner to corner.

2

Remove one eyelash strip from its packaging, and move it around between your palms to soften the strip.

3

Measure the strip against your own lashes to match where your own lashes begin and end. Trim any excess.

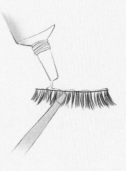

4

Once the lashes are cut to the perfect width and length, apply the glue evenly across the connecting strip directly from the tube.

5

Wait for about 60 seconds, until the glue becomes tacky, to get the lashes to stay in place more easily.

6

Using tweezers (or your fingers) place the strip on top of your natural lashes, at the lash root. Adjust the angle of the lashes to curl up at the ends for an open-eyed look, if desired.

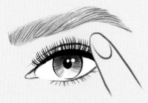

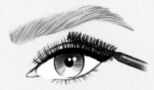

7

Hold the lashes against the skin of the inner corner and outer corner of the eye for a few seconds to get the lashes to bond.

8

When applying the second lash strip, be mindful to keep the angles of the lashes the same.

9

To fuse the false lash strip together visually with your natural lashes, apply mascara from the root of the lashes up to the tip.

> *TIP* • If one corner comes unstuck, add glue and hold the lashes in place for 15 seconds.

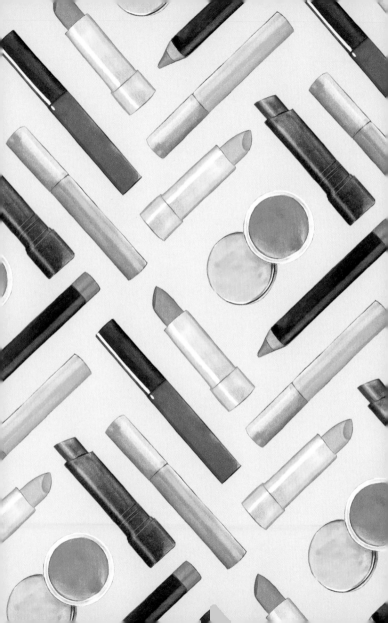

CHAPTER FOUR

LIPS

Fearless and wonderfully feminine, the impact of lip color lies entirely in how you wear it. Even fire-engine red can go classic, modern, and natural with variations in application.

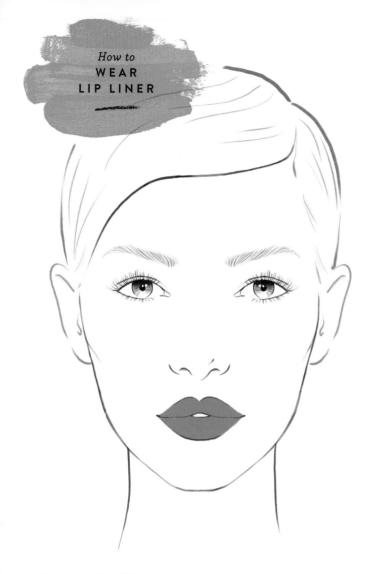

How to
WEAR
LIP LINER

The trick to locking any lip color in place is with the demarcating powers of lip liner.

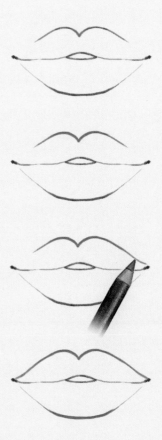

Start by defining your cupid's bow, the most complex part of your lip shape.

Trace the perimeter of your lips moving outward from the center.

Continue to the corner of your lips.

Starting at the center of your bottom lip, draw along the perimeter.

Connect the line all the way to the corners of your lip.

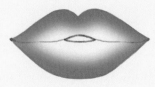

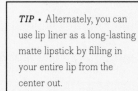

TIP • Blend the lip liner toward the center of your mouth for a more natural lipstick application.

TIP • Alternately, you can use lip liner as a long-lasting matte lipstick by filling in your entire lip from the center out.

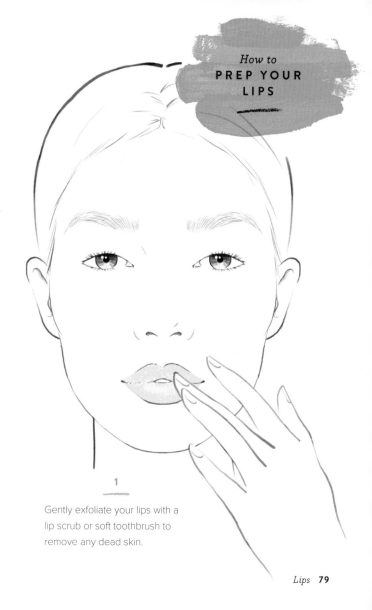

1

Gently exfoliate your lips with a
lip scrub or soft toothbrush to
remove any dead skin.

For a long-lasting lipstick that won't budge, smudge, or dry out your lips, start with these failsafe lip-smoothing and color-securing preparations.

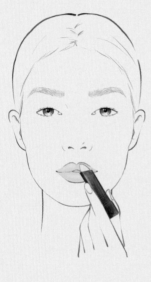

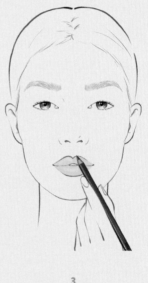

2

Apply a lip primer to enable longer wear for your lipstick.

3

Apply lip liner to the outer perimeter of the lips.

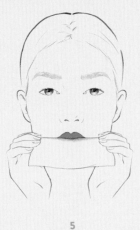

4

Apply lipstick.

Blot lipstick.

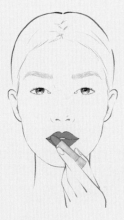

OPTIONAL: Apply translucent powder to lips for an extra-long-wear matte lipstick.

OPTIONAL: Apply an additional layer of lipstick.

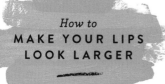

How to
MAKE YOUR LIPS
LOOK LARGER

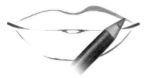

Starting at the center of the top lip, apply lip liner to the skin, following the outer perimeter of the lips.

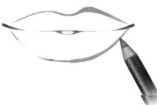

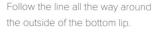
2

Follow the line all the way around the outside of the bottom lip.

3

Fill in lips with lipstick.

Pillowy lips can come by way of genetics or injections, but they can also be recreated with clever trompe l'oeil makeup.

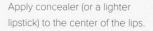

1

Apply lip balm or lipstick to lips.

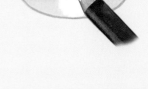

2

Apply concealer (or a lighter lipstick) to the center of the lips.

3

Blend the concealer (or lighter lipstick) out toward the sides of the lips with your fingers.

THE RULES OF LIP GLOSS

For the lipstick averse, lip gloss offers a hint of pigment without the commitment.

1

Apply an SPF-loaded lip balm first to avoid sun damage from light-catching gloss.

2

Sheer colors are easier to wear than opaque vinyl-finish colors, which can be difficult to keep in place.

3

Customize any lip gloss to your best shade by adding sheer lip balms like Elizabeth Arden Eight Hour Cream.

4

To get the finish you're looking for, follow this rule of thumb: the stickier the formula, the higher the shine.

To channel the high glamour of a Hollywood screen siren, six steps will achieve crisp, smudge-proof lines.

How to
GET PERFECT OLD-HOLLYWOOD LIPS

1

Using a color-matched lip liner, draw a diagonal line from one of the points of your cupid's bow down to the center of your top lip.

2

Crossing the first line, draw a diagonal line from the opposite tip of your cupid's bow down to the center of your top lip.

3

Following the perimeter of your bottom lip, draw a line along the center.

4

Place dots midway between the center edge of your lips and the corners of your lips.

5

Connect the dots.

6

Fill in your lips with lipstick.

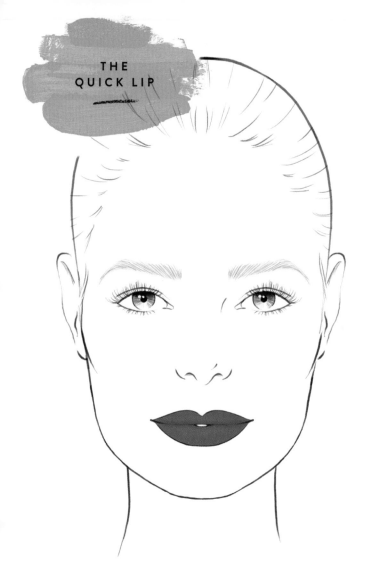

THE
QUICK LIP

Today's women don't have to overthink their lipstick application—
a quick daub of pigment with the fingers has a charm all its own.

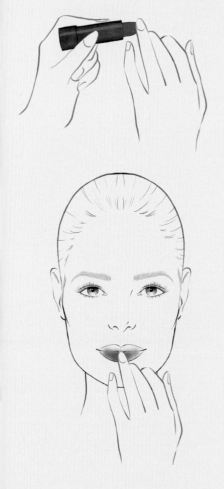

1

Apply lipstick onto your forefinger.

2

Smooth lipstick onto your lips with your finger.

3

Press lips together.

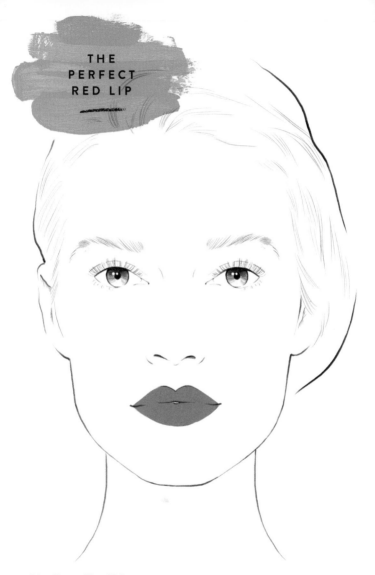

THE
PERFECT
RED LIP

A time-honored beauty tradition, a crimson lip is at once daring and romantic, and always individual.

1

Using a color-matched red lip liner, trace the perimeter of your cupid's bow from the center out.

2

Starting at the outer corners of the top lip, trace the perimeter of your upper lip to meet your first line.

3

Starting at the center of your bottom lip and extending to the corners of your mouth, complete the line on the border of your lip.

4

Using a brush, fill in your lips with lipstick.

5

Use a concealer brush and trace the outside of your lips with concealer to ensure your lipstick doesn't bleed.

6

Blend the concealer into your natural skin tone. (This will also make your lips look larger.)

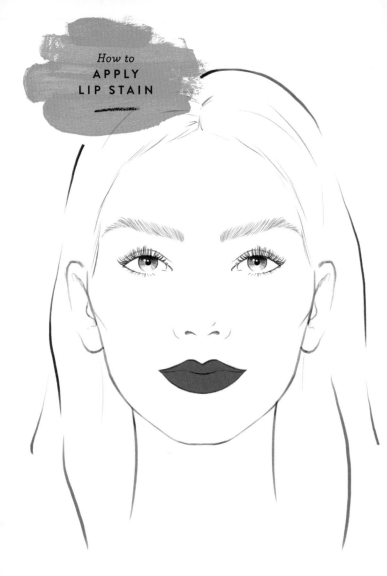

How to
**APPLY
LIP STAIN**

The most budge-proof of all lip colors, lip stains were invented to last well through the night.

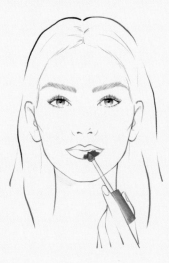

1

Apply lip stain to your whole bottom lip.

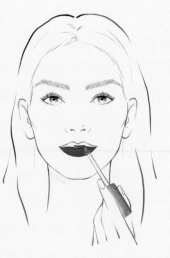

2

Apply a bit of lip stain to the center of your upper lip.

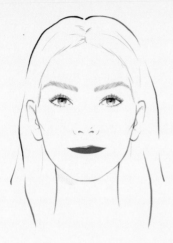

Press lips together.

4

Fill in any remaining negative space on your lips with color and blot.

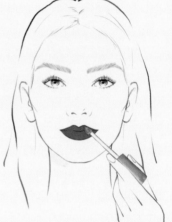

TIP • Most lip stains can do double duty as a cheek tint for an ultra-natural, blushing from-within look.

How to Choose

DARK LIPSTICK

From rich plums to gothic oxblood, dark lipstick is easily navigated with a two-part customizable blend.

1

Apply a cranberry lipstick

2

Add black lipstick until your desired shade is reached.

> **TIP** • Try this with emboldened brows and warm apricot blush.

NUDE LIPSTICK

Taking your lips from naked to next-level nude only requires finding the right shade to complement your complexion.

Fair skin tones can add warmth to the face with sheer baby-pink formulas.

Rosy-beige nudes complement light skin tones, which can also pull off a caramel-toned beige lipstick in a shade darker than their own skin.

Medium complexions are tonally suited for rosy lipsticks, in shades as dark or just lighter than the skin.

Deep skin tones go well with cinnamon-hued lip colors, especially those in a glossy formula.

Pink is the most ubiquitous lipstick color for its universally flattering properties. But, when specially tailored to your skin tone, it has the ability to brighten your whole look.

Fair faces can go in one of two directions: crisp neon-pink shades that pop against your pale backdrop, or soft peach-driven shades that help to neutralize unwanted redness in the skin.

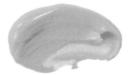

Light skin tones are best complemented by lipstick choices that are equally muted, such as sheer petal pinks.

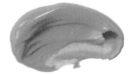

Medium complexions can balance almost any pink shade against their olivine undertones, but glowing yellow-based watermelons are a surefire win.

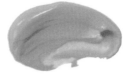

Deep skin tones can fearlessly experiment with blue-based fuchsias but should steer clear of neutral pale pinks, which will wash them out.

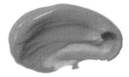

How to
APPLY
GRADIENT LIPS

Harnessing the charm of just-kissed lips or the remnants of summer popsicles, gradient lips concentrate pigment at the center of the mouth and are guaranteed to wear well.

1

Working quickly, apply lip stain to the center of your bottom lip, starting at its uppermost perimeter and going about halfway down.

2

Apply lip stain to the center of your top lip.

3

Before it has completely dried, blend the stain on your bottom lip out, but not all the way to the edge of your lips. Do the same to the top lip.

4

Apply lip balm for a seamless blend.

How to
SMOOTH LINES AROUND YOUR LIPS

When to
REAPPLY YOUR LIPSTICK

1

Trace along the edge of the lips with a transparent lip liner.

2

Apply concealer on the outside of your lip line.

3

Blend the concealer out with your fingertips.

The better preparation you give your lipstick, the less you'll have to think about it. But you may want to consider checking the state of your mouth…

1

After you finish a meal.

2

After you finish a beverage (when possible, use a straw).

3

In the middle of the day.

4

Before you go out for the night.

Where to STORE LIP BALM

1

Always keep one in your bag, so you never have to worry about not having it.

2

Stow one in your glove compartment, where it's out of the sun and within arm's reach.

3

Keep a trustworthy lip balm at your desk to reapply as often as necessary.

4

Pack one in your carry on—airplanes are extremely dehydrating. You'll be grateful to have one with you midflight.

5

Have an extra hydrating formula on your nightstand to apply before bed for overnight replenishment.

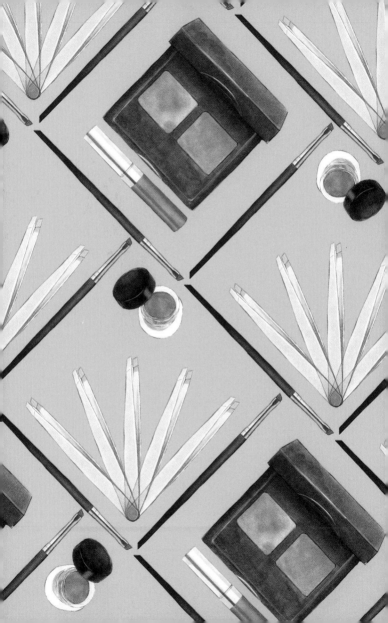

CHAPTER FIVE

EYEBROWS

From dramatically drawn on to bleached to nonexistent, eyebrows hold a lot of style and personality in a slim strip of hair. Between plucking, grooming, and filling in your brows, there are many ways to put a signature on what may be your most recognizable feature.

FIND THE BEST EYEBROWS FOR YOUR FACE SHAPE

While all eyebrows are individual, your face provides guidelines for shaping your own brows to best complement your natural bone structure.

Oval faces have easily balanced proportions and don't require exaggerated shapes. Instead, soft, angled eyebrows will frame them most naturally.

Long, rectangular faces will find that straight eyebrows with little to no arch help balance high foreheads and cheekbones.

Round faces will gain visual length and definition from more sharply arched brows.

Heart-shaped faces will find an ideal eyebrow in softly rounded shapes.

Square faces with strong jawlines can carry a softly arched brow, to soften the lines of the face.

Diamond-shaped faces are better suited for dramatically curved arches to refocus attention on the narrow parts of the face like the forehead.

How to FIND THE RIGHT EYEBROW COLOR

To fill in your eyebrows in the most natural way possible, always choose a tone a bit cooler than your own brow hair color.

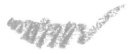

VERY LIGHT
Barely there blondes should look for ashy-gray eyebrow pencils and powders.

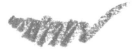

DARK
For medium- and dark-brown brows, a deep, cool brown will make the most natural accompaniment.

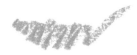

LIGHT
Golden blondes can embolden their brows with cool beige tones.

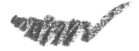

VERY DARK
Black and nearly black hair can be filled in with an almost-black pigment.

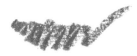

MEDIUM
Light brunettes should reach for a midrange brown, a color that will very subtly strengthen medium brunette arches.

How to
PLUCK YOUR EYEBROWS

3

To find your natural arch without placing it too close to the inside of your brow, looking straight forward, line your tweezers or pencil from the outside of your nostril to the outside of your pupil. Your arch should rest where the tweezers hit at your brow bone. Avoid overplucking hair below the arches—they will look unnatural.

4

To find the point where your eyebrows should end, line your tweezers or pencil from the outside of your nostril to the outer corner of your eye. Your eyebrow should stop where your tweezers hit at your brow bone. Very little hair should be plucked from the ends of the eyebrow.

TIP • Tweezing after the shower, when your pores are open, will allow for easier and less painful hair removal.

1

In good lighting, hold skin taught and pull hairs in the direction of growth. Use tweezers with sharp, slanted edges.

2

To find where your eyebrows should start, line your tweezers or pencil vertically from the outer edge of your nostril to the inner corner of your eye. Your eyebrows should start where the tweezers hit at your brow bone. Do the same on the opposite side. Tweeze errant hairs between your brows.

What to Do About

THIN EYEBROWS

Worn by screen sirens like Greta Garbo and nineties waifs like Kate Moss, the skinny brow has its appeal. But those looking to reverse the results of accidental overplucking will find that allowing their eyebrows to grow out for a period of three to four months will help them find their natural shape and arch again.

THICK EYEBROWS

Congratulations, according to the zeitgeist, you've won the genetic jackpot. Simply combing your brows will do wonders for unruly arches, as will plucking a few errant hairs—not every woman is bold enough to lean into a full-fledged unibrow.

STRAIGHT EYEBROWS

Despite popular opinion, dramatically arched eyebrows are not suited to every face. Simply look to the likes of Rooney Mara and Audrey Hepburn as your guide—straight brows are even more becoming when they're emboldened.

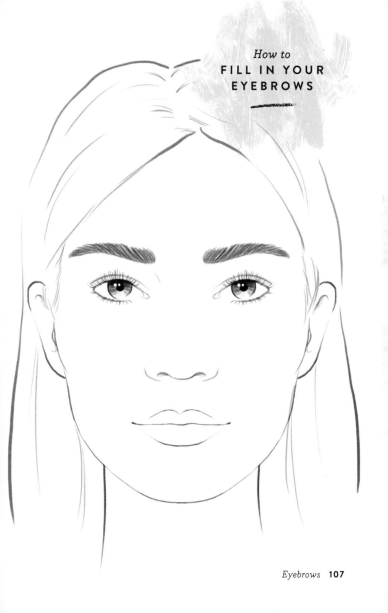

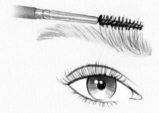

1

Brush your brows up.

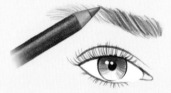

2

Using an eyebrow pencil, draw hair-like strokes starting at the base of the brow and going up.

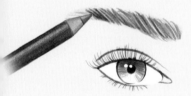

3

Continue to the outer part of the eyebrow, drawing strokes out following the natural direction of your hair.

4

If necessary, lightly fill in any spare space in the inner corners of your brow to naturally blend with the rest of your brow.

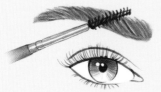

Comb through your eyebrows
with a spoolie or eyebrow brush
to blend.

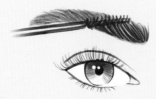

6

Set the look and direction of
your eyebrows with a clear or
tinted eyebrow gel.

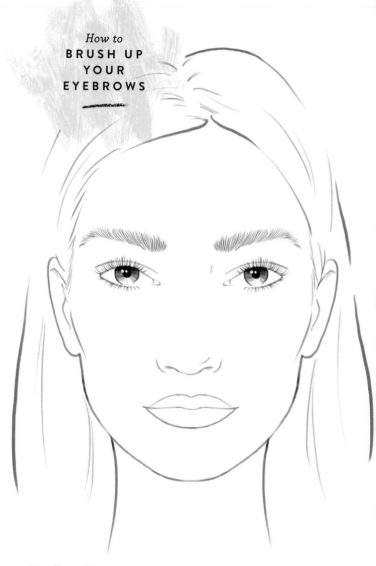

How to
**BRUSH UP
YOUR
EYEBROWS**

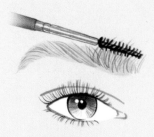

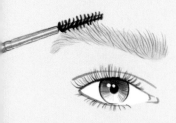

Using clear or tinted eyebrow gel, brush your hair up at the beginning of your brows (closest to the nose), continuing to comb your hair up and out toward your arches. Finally, brush the ends of your eyebrows out toward your temples.

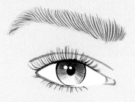

> *TIP* • For a more feral look, brush all parts of your eyebrows as straight up as possible.

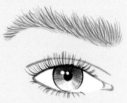

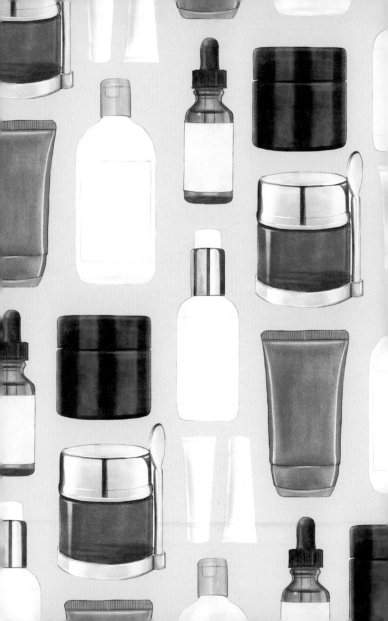

SKINCARE

*No amount of makeup can replicate
the power of a good complexion.
When you have great skin, makeup
becomes a playful accessory, not a
necessity.*

How to
REMOVE
MAKEUP

When wearing makeup, especially a base, bronzer, or blush, always be sure to clean it from your face. Taking it off is as simple as finding the right makeup remover.

1

Saturate a cotton pad with cleansing water, coconut oil, a gel-based makeup remover, or a milky cleanser, and gently use it to wipe the majority of makeup from your face. Use both sides of the pad.

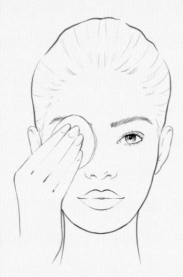

Saturate a second cotton pad with your makeup remover of choice (see previous step) and gently swipe it from the inner corner of your eye outward. For extra-heavy eye makeup, start by pressing the saturated pad on your closed lid for a few seconds before wiping.

3

Use an additional saturated cotton pad to wipe lipstick off your lips. For especially long-wearing formulas, apply petroleum jelly or coconut oil to your lips and let it sit for a few minutes, then gently buff off the lipstick with a warm washcloth, working in a circular motion.

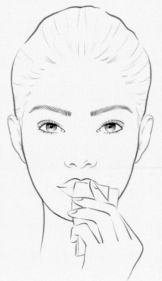

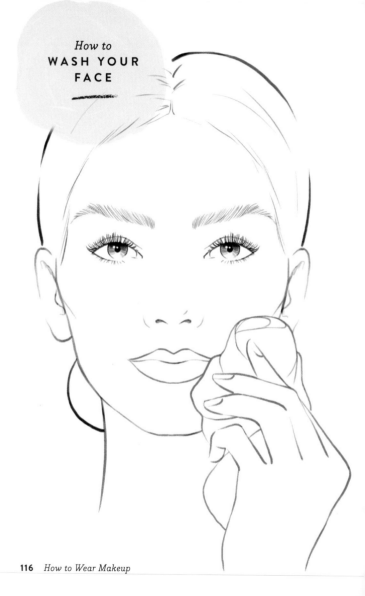

How to
WASH YOUR FACE

It is among the cardinal sins in beauty to not wash your face before falling asleep. Cleansing is an important ritual for the beginning of your skincare routine.

1

Splash tepid water on your face.

2

Put a quarter-size amount of cleanser on your fingers and rub your hands together.

3

Massage the cleanser in a zig-zagging motion (up and down) across your forehead.

4

Massage the cleanser down the bridge of your nose and out across the cheeks toward your ears.

5

Follow the jawline starting at the center of your chin and going up to your ears, massaging the cleanser into your skin.

6

Splash tepid water on your face until the cleanser is completely washed off. Repeat if necessary.

7

Pat—don't rub—your skin dry with a clean towel.

> *TIP* • Most cleansers will target a skin type directly on the label. But acne-prone skin types can opt for formulas with salicylic acid or honey, which is antibacterial. Oily skin should reach for oil-free gel-based formulas. Combination skin can use anything so long as it's not too drying. Dry skin types should use milk, cream, or oil-based cleansers. Sensitive skin should look for gentle cleansers with few ingredients.

How to Use

FACE MIST

One of the most pleasurable aspects of skincare, face mists are designed to give you instant, on-the-go hydration that is all but guaranteed to elevate your mood and energy. But a spritz of face mist can also work as a skincare primer, contributing a thin, easily absorbable layer of moisture to your skin before you layer on moisturizer. And, even better, a quick mist will give cakey-looking makeup a lived-in finish.

TONER

Classically designed to reestablish the pH balance of your skin and to remove any excess dirt or makeup that your cleanser missed, modern toners are now formulated to also prevent breakouts, counter dryness, and add an extra boost of complexion-brightening ingredients to your skin. After washing your face, apply your toner to a cotton pad and press onto dry skin.

How to
USE SERUMS

Created to target your primary skin concerns, from dullness to acne and aging, serums are denser with active nutrients than your average moisturizer. Apply after washing (or using toner) and wear alone or layer under moisturizer.

ANTI-AGING

Look for serums packed with pollution- and UV-fighting antioxidants, such as vitamin C. Peptides and growth factors will also strengthen the skin against wrinkles.

LIFTED APPEARANCE

Peptides boost collagen and elastin production to restore strength to the skin for a firmer, tighter look.

BRIGHTER COMPLEXION

Retinol and vitamin A are ingredients that will accelerate cell renewal to smooth the complexion and make the skin more radiant.

APPLY EYE CREAM

The skin bordering your eye is surprisingly idiosyncratic. Targeted creams address the especially delicate skin, small pores, and dark circles surrounding the eye.

1

Dot on your eye cream along the lowest border of your under-eye area. Don't get too close to the eyes.

2

Gently press the eye cream into your skin with your ring finger, outside to inside, to avoid tugging the skin and causing future wrinkles.

3

Spread any remaining product under your brow bone.

4

End with a gentle circular motion, starting at the inner brow bone, working out to the outer brow bone, down to the outer corner of your under eye, and in to the inner corner.

How to
MOISTURIZE
THE RIGHT WAY

Moisturizing is arguably the most important step in maintaining a radiant and wrinkle-free complexion.

1

Place a dime- to quarter-size amount of product in your hands, and warm it between your palms.

2

Gently press the product evenly into the face and neck.

3

Then start massaging into the jawline and chin with small, upward movements. Do not pull the skin.

4

Press the face cream into your cheeks, then onto your forehead.

5

Press remaining product onto your neck and décolletage.

How to
CHOOSE SUNSCREEN

The importance of daily sunscreen cannot be stressed enough for keeping your skin safe from premature aging and cancer-causing UV rays. Always choose a broad-spectrum formula with an SPF between 30 and 50—any lower will not be effective and any higher than 50 offers no added protection.

PHYSICAL

Zinc oxide and titanium dioxide are natural minerals that, when ground to a fine powder, block harmful rays from touching your skin. Generally speaking, these formulas tend to have a heavier feeling but a longer life on the skin than their chemical counterparts.

CHEMICAL

Chemical sunscreens block UV rays with carbon-compound cocktails that reduce ultraviolet radiation penetration to the skin, and can also contain UVB- and UVA-absorbing chemicals. They tend to have a lighter finish on the skin.

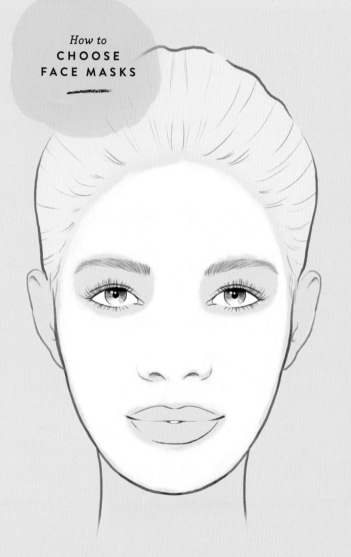

Supercharge your skincare routine with masks that help to hydrate, smooth fine lines, clear clogged pores, and boost radiance.

DETOX AND ACNE

Mud masks and charcoal-based masks draw impurities to the surface and deeply cleanse the skin.

RADIANCE

Chemical peels and physical exfoliating masks slough away dead skin cells for brighter-looking skin.

FINE LINES

Retinol masks and masks containing vitamin C and lactic acid will boost collagen production to reduce fine lines and wrinkles.

HYDRATE

Sheet masks, sleeping packs, hyaluronic acid masks, and moisture-rich masks will all help restore suppleness and glow to your skin.

DE-PUFFING

Cooling ingredients and caffeine will help boost circulation to de-puff the skin.

How to
MASSAGE YOUR FACE

Turn your daily skincare routine into an at-home spa treatment by applying serums and creams in a wrinkle-fighting, de-puffing, circulation-boosting face massage.

1

Using your fingertips, gently massage product from the lower neck upward to the chin.

2

Massage serum, cream, or sunscreen from the lower jaw to the earlobe. Repeat on the other side.

3

Massage from the chin to the earlobe. Repeat on other side.

4

In sweeping, gentle gestures, massage from the outer corner of your lips, under the cheekbone, up and out to your earlobe. Repeat on other side.

5

Massage the product from the outside of the nostril up to the temple. Repeat on other side.

6

Starting at the bottom outside of the nostril, massage up and in to the bridge of the nose.

7

Starting at the forehead and going up to the hairline, massage the product into forehead.

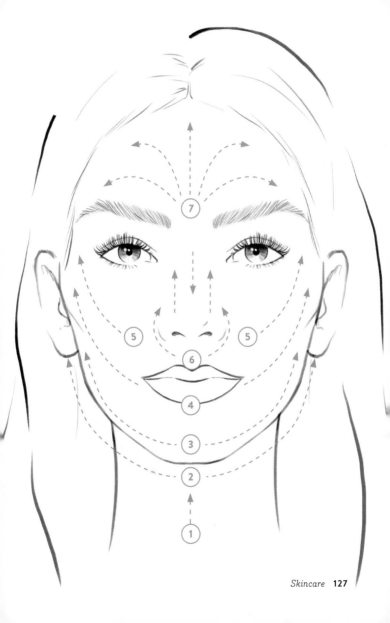

Editor: Camaren Subhiyah
Production Manager: Alex Cameron

Library of Congress Control Number: 2016949532

ISBN: 978-1-4197-2397-1

Printed and bound in China
10 9 8 7 6 5 4 3 2 1

Abrams books are available at special discounts when purchased
in quantity for premiums and promotions as well as fundraising
or educational use. Special editions can also be created to
specification. For details, contact specialsales@abramsbooks.com
or the address below.

ABRAMS The Art of Books
115 West 18th Street, New York, NY 10011
abramsbooks.com